STROKE DIET COOKBOOK

FOOD LIST

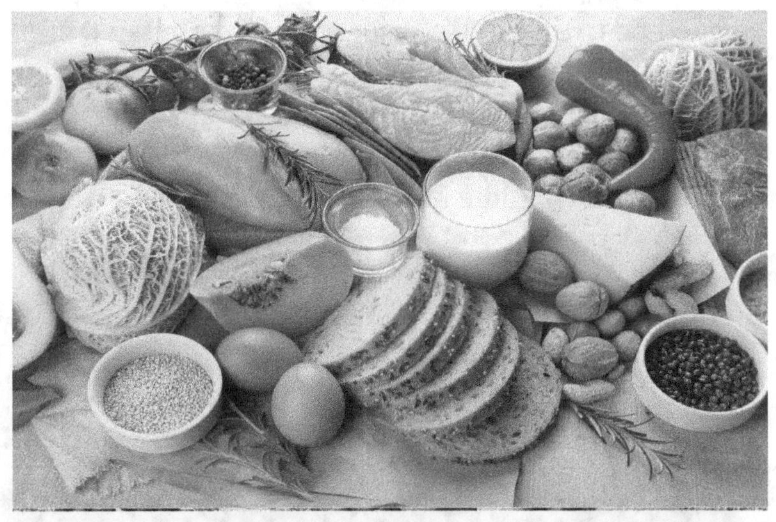

The Complete Guide to Managing Stroke Recovery with Comprehensive Food Lists, Meal Plans, and Recipes

Eddie M.Richards

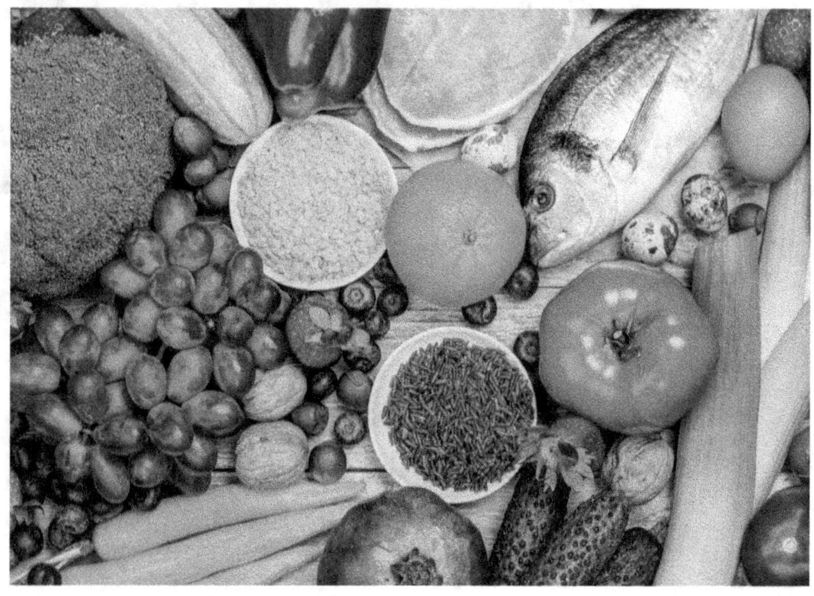

Table of Contents

Part 1: Introduction to the Stroke Diet

A stroke is a life-changing event, and the path to recovery requires a multifaceted approach. While medical intervention plays a crucial role, what you put on your plate can significantly impact your healing journey. This first section of our guide delves into the world of the stroke diet, equipping you with the knowledge and tools to make informed dietary choices that promote optimal recovery.

Chapter 1: Understanding Stroke Recovery and the Role of Diet

This chapter lays the groundwork by explaining the recovery process after a stroke. You'll gain insights into how different parts of the brain are affected and how the right nutrients can support their repair and function. We'll also explore the role of diet in managing risk factors like high blood pressure and cholesterol, often associated with stroke.

Chapter 2: The Science Behind the Stroke Diet - How Food Impacts Healing

This chapter delves deeper into the science behind the stroke diet. We'll explore how specific nutrients like vitamins, minerals, and antioxidants contribute to healing. You'll learn how certain foods can improve blood flow to the brain, reduce inflammation, and support the growth of new nerve cells.

Chapter 3: Benefits of Following a Stroke Diet

Following a stroke diet isn't just about restrictions; it's about unlocking a world of benefits for your recovery. This chapter dives into the tangible advantages you can expect. We'll discuss how the stroke diet can:

* Enhance cognitive function and memory
* Improve physical strength and mobility
* Reduce fatigue and boost energy levels
* Promote emotional well-being and mood
* Lower the risk of future strokes

By understanding these benefits, you'll be empowered to make conscious choices about the food you eat, becoming an active participant in your recovery.

Chapter 1: Understanding Stroke Recovery and the Role of Diet

A stroke disrupts the normal flow of blood to the brain, causing brain cells to die. The severity of a stroke depends on the location and size of the affected area. Recovery following a stroke is a remarkable process where the brain attempts to heal itself. This chapter explores how stroke recovery works and how the right diet can significantly impact this journey.

The Path to Recovery:

Following a stroke, the brain undergoes a process called neuroplasticity. This amazing ability allows undamaged brain areas to take over functions previously handled by the damaged region. The more you stimulate these healthy areas, the stronger these new connections become. Rehabilitation therapies, including physical, occupational, and speech therapy, play a crucial role in stimulating these pathways and promoting functional recovery.

Fueling the Healing Process:

Just like a car needs the right fuel to run efficiently, your brain requires specific nutrients to support healing and neuroplasticity. The food you eat provides the building blocks for repairing damaged cells, fostering the growth of new connections, and optimizing brain function.

Key Nutrients for Stroke Recovery:

This chapter will delve into some of the key nutrients crucial for stroke recovery:

* Omega-3 Fatty Acids: Found in fatty fish, flaxseeds, and walnuts, these fats play a vital role in reducing inflammation and promoting cognitive function.

* Antioxidants: Present in fruits, vegetables, and whole grains, antioxidants combat free radicals, which can damage brain cells after a stroke.

* Protein: Essential for building and repairing tissues, protein is vital for muscle recovery and overall well-being. Lean protein sources like chicken, fish, and beans are excellent choices.

* B Vitamins: These vitamins are crucial for neurological function and energy production.

Whole grains, leafy greens, and legumes are rich sources of B vitamins.

Diet and Risk Factor Management:

Stroke is often linked to pre-existing health conditions like high blood pressure, high cholesterol, and diabetes. A well-designed stroke diet can help manage these risk factors by:

* Limiting Saturated and Trans Fats: These fats contribute to high cholesterol levels, increasing the risk of stroke.

* Controlling Sodium Intake: Excessive sodium can lead to high blood pressure, a major risk factor for stroke.

* Managing Blood Sugar: If you have diabetes, the stroke diet can help regulate blood sugar levels, reducing the risk of complications.

By understanding the connection between diet and stroke recovery, you can make informed dietary choices that empower your healing journey.

Chapter 2: The Science Behind the Stroke Diet - How Food Impacts Healing

A stroke disrupts the delicate balance of the brain, impacting its ability to function optimally. While medications and therapy play a crucial role in recovery, the food you choose can significantly influence the healing process at a cellular level. This chapter delves into the science behind the stroke diet, exploring how specific nutrients contribute to a successful recovery.

The Power of Nutrients:

The human body is a complex ecosystem, and the food we eat provides the building blocks for cellular processes. After a stroke, damaged brain cells require specific nutrients to support repair and regeneration. Let's explore some key players in the stroke recovery symphony:

* Antioxidants: Imagine tiny shields protecting brain cells from free radicals – harmful molecules produced during the body's natural processes and by external factors like stress. Fruits and vegetables are powerhouses of antioxidants like vitamins C and E, beta-carotene, and lycopene. These

antioxidants neutralize free radicals, minimizing damage to brain cells and fostering a healthy environment for healing.

* Omega-3 Fatty Acids: Often referred to as "brain food," omega-3 fatty acids play a critical role in reducing inflammation, a common outcome after a stroke. Inflammation can hinder the healing process, and omega-3s, found in fatty fish, flaxseeds, and walnuts, work to combat this inflammatory response. Studies suggest omega-3s may also enhance cognitive function and memory.

* Neurotrophic Factors: These are special molecules that act like fertilizers for the brain, stimulating the growth and development of new nerve cells. A stroke can damage existing nerve connections and hinder the formation of new ones. Foods rich in B vitamins, particularly B12 and folic acid, found in leafy greens, legumes, and fortified cereals, can support the production of neurotrophic factors, promoting the creation of new neural pathways for optimal recovery.

* Blood Flow Boosters: Proper blood flow is essential for delivering oxygen and nutrients to the brain. Nitric oxide, a molecule that helps relax blood vessels and improve blood flow, can be

stimulated by consuming foods rich in L-arginine, an amino acid found in red meat, poultry, nuts, and seeds. Improved blood flow ensures proper delivery of vital nutrients to the healing brain.

Beyond Individual Nutrients:

While individual nutrients play crucial roles, the magic truly happens when they work synergistically. A balanced stroke diet rich in a variety of fruits, vegetables, whole grains, lean protein, and healthy fats provides a comprehensive array of nutrients to support the complex healing process after a stroke.

Optimizing Brain Function:

The right diet can go beyond supporting cellular repair. Studies suggest that certain nutrients, like flavonoids found in fruits like berries, may enhance cognitive function and memory. Additionally, a healthy diet can improve mood and reduce fatigue, common challenges faced after a stroke.

By understanding the science behind the stroke diet, you can become an active participant in your recovery, making conscious food choices that empower your brain to heal and thrive.

Chapter 3: Benefits of Following a Stroke Diet

A stroke disrupts your life, but it doesn't have to define your future. Following a stroke diet isn't just about restrictions; it's a powerful tool to actively participate in your recovery and unlock a world of benefits. This chapter dives into the tangible ways a well-designed stroke diet can enhance your journey back to health.

Boosting Brain Power:

* Enhanced Cognitive Function and Memory: The stroke diet provides the brain with the building blocks it needs to repair damaged cells and foster the growth of new connections. This can lead to improved cognitive function, memory, and concentration, allowing you to regain clarity and focus.

* Sharper Thinking and Processing: A balanced stroke diet rich in omega-3 fatty acids and antioxidants can improve blood flow to the brain, delivering vital oxygen and nutrients. This enhanced circulation promotes sharper thinking, quicker processing, and better problem-solving abilities.

Regaining Physical Strength and Mobility:

* Improved Muscle Recovery: Protein is a critical nutrient for rebuilding and repairing tissues, including muscles. The stroke diet emphasizes lean protein sources, aiding in muscle recovery and helping you regain strength and mobility. This is crucial for regaining independence and performing daily activities with ease.

* Increased Energy Levels: A stroke can leave you feeling fatigued. The stroke diet focuses on complex carbohydrates and healthy fats, providing sustained energy throughout the day. This allows you to participate actively in rehabilitation therapies and engage in daily life with renewed vigor.

Emotional and Mental Well-being:

* Reduced Fatigue and Improved Mood: Following a stroke diet can combat fatigue by providing a steady stream of energy. Additionally, certain nutrients may influence mood regulation, helping to combat feelings of depression or anxiety that can sometimes occur after a stroke.

* Enhanced Sleep Quality: A balanced diet rich in essential nutrients promotes healthy sleep patterns. This allows your body and brain to rest and repair more effectively, contributing to overall well-being.

Long-Term Health Benefits:

* Lower Risk of Future Strokes: By managing risk factors like high blood pressure, high cholesterol, and diabetes, the stroke diet can significantly reduce the risk of experiencing another stroke in the future.

* Improved Overall Health: The principles of a stroke diet – emphasizing fruits, vegetables, whole grains, and lean protein – promote overall health and wellness. This translates to a stronger immune system, improved cardiovascular health, and a reduced risk of chronic diseases.

Investing in Yourself:

Following a stroke diet is an investment in your most valuable asset – your health. By making informed dietary choices, you empower your body and brain to heal optimally. The benefits go beyond physical recovery, promoting emotional well-being and a renewed sense of vitality. This chapter concludes by encouraging you to discuss your individual needs with a healthcare professional or registered dietitian who can create a personalized stroke diet plan to unlock your full recovery potential.

Part 2: Foundation of the Stroke Diet

Building a strong foundation is crucial for any successful endeavor, and the stroke diet is no exception. This section delves into the essential food groups that form the bedrock of a healthy and recovery-promoting diet after a stroke. We'll also explore foods to limit or avoid to optimize your healing journey.

Chapter 4: Essential Food Groups for Stroke Recovery

A well-balanced stroke diet incorporates a variety of nutrient-rich food groups, each playing a vital role in the recovery process. Here, we'll explore these key groups in detail:

* Fruits and Vegetables: A Rainbow of Nutrients: These vibrant powerhouses are brimming with antioxidants, vitamins, minerals, and fiber. Antioxidants protect brain cells from damage, while vitamins and minerals support various functions crucial for healing. Fiber keeps you feeling full and promotes healthy digestion. Aim for a variety of

colorful fruits and vegetables throughout the day to reap the benefits of a diverse range of nutrients.

* Whole Grains: Filling Up on Fiber and Power: Whole grains provide sustained energy through complex carbohydrates, keeping you feeling fuller for longer. They are also a rich source of fiber, which aids digestion and helps manage blood sugar levels. Opt for brown rice, quinoa, whole-wheat bread and pasta, and oats to incorporate this essential group into your stroke diet.

* Lean Protein: Building and Repairing Body Tissue: Protein is the building block of life, and after a stroke, it's vital for repairing damaged tissues and promoting muscle recovery. Lean protein sources like chicken, fish, beans, lentils, and tofu provide essential amino acids without the added saturated fat often found in red meat.

* Low-Fat Dairy: Strengthening Bones and Immunity: Low-fat dairy products like milk, yogurt, and cheese offer a good source of calcium and vitamin D, crucial for bone health and overall well-being. Additionally, yogurt provides probiotics, which can benefit gut health and immunity. Opt for low-fat or fat-free options to minimize saturated fat intake.

* Healthy Fats: Fueling the Brain and Body:
Healthy fats, particularly omega-3 fatty acids found
in fatty fish, flaxseeds, and walnuts, play a critical
role in reducing inflammation and promoting
cognitive function. Additionally, healthy fats
provide sustained energy and contribute to a feeling
of satiety.

Chapter 5: Foods to Limit or Avoid After a Stroke

While certain foods are beneficial for stroke
recovery, others can hinder progress. This chapter
delves into foods to limit or avoid to optimize your
healing journey:

* Saturated and Trans Fats: These fats raise
unhealthy cholesterol levels, increasing the risk of
stroke and heart disease. Limit processed foods,
fried foods, fatty meats, and full-fat dairy products.

* Added Sugar: While some natural sugars in fruits
are beneficial, added sugars found in sugary drinks,
desserts, and processed snacks contribute to weight
gain and can lead to blood sugar spikes. Opt for
naturally sweet fruits and limit added sugars.

* Sodium: Excessive sodium intake can raise blood pressure, a significant risk factor for stroke. Limit processed foods, canned goods, and added table salt. Explore flavorful herbs and spices to add taste to your dishes.

Remember: This is a general guideline, and your specific needs may vary. It's crucial to consult with your healthcare professional or registered dietitian to create a personalized stroke diet plan tailored to your unique situation and medical history.

Chapter 4: Essential Food Groups for Stroke Recovery

Following a stroke, your body enters a remarkable healing phase. To support this process, you need a diet rich in a variety of nutrients, each playing a specific role in your recovery journey. This chapter explores the five essential food groups that form the foundation of a stroke-friendly diet:

1. Fruits and Vegetables: A Rainbow of Antioxidants and Vitality

Imagine a vibrant garden overflowing with life – that's the essence of incorporating fruits and vegetables into your stroke diet. These powerhouses are packed with antioxidants, which act as shields for your brain cells, protecting them from damage caused by free radicals.

* Antioxidant All-Stars: Fruits like berries, oranges, kiwi, and vegetables like leafy greens, broccoli, bell peppers, and tomatoes are brimming with antioxidants like vitamins C and E, beta-carotene, and lycopene.

Benefits Beyond Protection:

Fruits and vegetables are more than just antioxidant powerhouses. They are excellent sources of essential vitamins and minerals like:

* Vitamin K: Crucial for blood clotting, which becomes even more important after a stroke. Leafy greens like kale and spinach are rich sources of vitamin K.

* Potassium: Helps regulate blood pressure, a key factor in preventing future strokes. Fruits like bananas and cantaloupe are good sources of potassium.

* Fiber: Keeps you feeling full and promotes healthy digestion. Fruits with skin like apples and pears, and vegetables like Brussels sprouts and artichokes are high in fiber.

Variety is Key:

Don't settle for a monotonous diet! Aim for a rainbow of colors on your plate. Each color represents a unique set of phytonutrients, offering a broader spectrum of health benefits.

Tips for Inclusion:

* Start your day with a smoothie packed with fruits
and vegetables.
* Add chopped vegetables to omelet or scrambled
eggs for breakfast.
* Snack on fruits and baby carrots throughout the
day.
* Include roasted vegetables as a side dish with
dinner.

2. Whole Grains: Fueling Your Body for Recovery

Whole grains are the unsung heroes of a stroke diet.
They are complex carbohydrates, providing
sustained energy throughout the day, unlike simple
carbohydrates found in sugary foods that can lead
to energy crashes.

Fiber Power: Whole grains are packed with fiber,
which offers a multitude of benefits:

* Aids Digestion: Fiber helps your digestive system
function smoothly, preventing constipation, a
common concern after a stroke.

* Manages Blood Sugar: Fiber slows down the
absorption of sugar into the bloodstream, helping
to regulate blood sugar levels.

* Promotes Satiety: Fiber keeps you feeling fuller for longer, reducing cravings and aiding in weight management.

Whole Grain Choices:

Swap refined grains like white bread and pasta for their whole-grain counterparts. Here are some excellent choices:

* Brown Rice: A versatile grain that can be enjoyed in main dishes and salads.

* Quinoa: A complete protein source offering a nutty flavor and a fluffy texture.

* Whole-Wheat Bread and Pasta: Choose whole-wheat options for sandwiches and pasta dishes.

* Oats: A heart-healthy breakfast option rich in soluble fiber.

3. Lean Protein: Building and Repairing Tissue

After a stroke, your body enters a rebuilding phase, and protein is the essential building block for repairing damaged tissues and promoting muscle recovery. Lean protein sources provide amino acids, the building blocks of protein, without excess saturated fat.

Choosing Wisely:

Opt for lean protein sources like:

* Chicken and Turkey: Excellent sources of protein with minimal fat content. Choose skinless, boneless options for the healthiest preparation.

* Fish: Fatty fish like salmon, tuna, and mackerel are rich in omega-3 fatty acids, crucial for brain health. Aim for at least two servings of fish per week.

* Beans and Lentils: Plant-based protein sources packed with fiber and essential nutrients. They are also a budget-friendly option.

* Tofu and Tempeh: Soy-based protein options that are versatile and can be incorporated into various dishes.

Spread the Protein Throughout the Day:

Don't limit protein to just dinner. Include it in every meal and snack to ensure your body has a continuous supply of amino acids for repair and recovery.

4. Low-Fat Dairy: Strengthening Bones and Immunity

Low-fat dairy products offer a valuable source of calcium and vitamin D, both vital for bone health and overall well-being.

* Calcium: Plays a crucial role in maintaining strong bones, which is especially important after a stroke to prevent fractures.

* Vitamin D: Aids in calcium absorption and supports immune function.

Focus on Low-Fat Options:

Choose low-fat or fat-free milk, yogurt, and cheese to minimize saturated fat intake. Here are some tips for incorporating low-fat dairy into your stroke diet:

* Start your day with a protein smoothie made with low-fat yogurt, berries, and a scoop of protein powder.

* Enjoy a cup of low-fat milk or fortified plant-based milk with your breakfast cereal.

* Incorporate low-fat yogurt with fruit and granola for a midday snack.

* Use low-fat shredded cheese sparingly on salads or baked potatoes.

* Experiment with low-fat cottage cheese as a protein topping for whole-wheat toast.

5. Healthy Fats: Fueling the Brain and Body

Not all fats are created equal. While saturated and trans fats can be detrimental to health, healthy fats play a crucial role in stroke recovery.

* Omega-3 Power: Omega-3 fatty acids found in fatty fish like salmon, tuna, and mackerel, as well as flaxseeds and walnuts, are essential for reducing inflammation and promoting cognitive function. Aim for at least two servings of fatty fish per week.

* Benefits Beyond Omega-3s: Healthy fats also contribute to:

* Feeling Full: They promote satiety, helping you manage your weight and avoid unhealthy snacking.

* Nutrient Absorption: Certain vitamins, like vitamin A, are fat-soluble, meaning they require fat for proper absorption.

Making Smart Choices:

Incorporate healthy fats into your diet by:

* Drizzling olive oil over salads or vegetables.
* Using avocado slices on toast or sandwiches.
* Adding a handful of nuts or seeds to yogurt or oatmeal.

Remember:

* Balance is key. While healthy fats are beneficial, moderation is important.
* Consult a healthcare professional or registered dietitian for personalized guidance on incorporating healthy fats into your stroke diet.

By incorporating these essential food groups into your daily meals, you'll be providing your body with the necessary nutrients to support optimal healing and recovery after a stroke. The next chapter will

explore foods to limit or avoid to further optimize
your journey back to health.

Chapter 5: Foods to Limit or Avoid After a Stroke - Optimizing Your Recovery Journey

A stroke disrupts the normal functioning of the body, and certain dietary choices can hinder your healing process. This chapter delves into foods to limit or avoid after a stroke, allowing you to make informed decisions that promote optimal recovery.

Limiting Saturated and Trans Fats:

Saturated and trans fats are the villains in a stroke-friendly diet. They contribute to high LDL ("bad") cholesterol levels, increasing the risk of stroke and other cardiovascular diseases. Here's why it's crucial to limit these fats:

* Clogged Arteries: Saturated fat promotes the buildup of plaque in your arteries, narrowing the pathways for blood flow to the brain. This can increase the risk of future strokes.

* Inflammation Boosters: Trans fats, found in processed foods like fried foods, baked goods, and margarine, contribute to inflammation throughout the body, which can hinder healing after a stroke.

Where to Find Them:

Be mindful of these hidden culprits:

* Fatty meats: Limit red meat like beef and pork, and choose leaner options like chicken or turkey without the skin.

* Processed meats: Avoid sausages, hot dogs, bacon, and deli meats, which are often loaded with saturated fat and sodium.

* Fried foods: Opt for baked, grilled, or steamed cooking methods instead of frying, which adds saturated fat and trans fats.

* Pastries and baked goods: Limit commercially prepared pastries, cakes, cookies, and doughnuts that are often high in unhealthy fats and added sugars.

Making Smart Swaps:

* Replace fatty cuts of meat with fish, especially those rich in omega-3 fatty acids, which offer heart-healthy benefits.
* Choose lean protein sources like beans, lentils, and tofu for a plant-based alternative.

* Cook with heart-healthy oils like olive oil or avocado oil instead of butter or lard.
* Opt for whole-wheat bread and baked goods made with minimal saturated fat.

Sodium: Mind Your Salt Intake:

Sodium is an essential mineral, but excessive intake can be detrimental after a stroke. Here's why managing sodium is crucial:

* Blood Pressure Booster: High sodium intake contributes to elevated blood pressure, a significant risk factor for stroke.

* Fluid Retention: Excessive sodium can cause fluid retention, putting extra strain on the heart and circulatory system.

Where Does It Hide?

Be aware of these common sources of high sodium:

* Processed foods: Canned goods, frozen meals, packaged snacks, and condiments are often loaded with sodium. Read labels carefully and choose low-sodium options.

* Added table salt: Limit your use of salt when cooking and avoid adding it at the table. Explore flavorful herbs and spices to add taste to your food.

* Restaurant meals: Restaurant food is notorious for being high in sodium. Choose grilled or baked options and request sauces and dressings on the side.

Making Smart Choices:

* Cook more meals at home, allowing you to control the sodium content.
* Rinse canned vegetables to remove some of the sodium before adding them to your dish.
* Choose fresh or frozen vegetables with "no added salt" labels.
* Opt for low-sodium broths and soups.

Added Sugar: Friend or Foe in Stroke Recovery?

Sugar provides energy, but added sugars found in processed foods and sugary drinks can be detrimental after a stroke. Here's why moderation is key:

* Blood Sugar Spikes: Added sugars can cause blood sugar spikes and crashes, leading to fatigue and difficulty concentrating.

* Weight Gain: Excessive sugar intake can contribute to weight gain, increasing the risk of complications like diabetes, which can further impact heart health.

Where Does It Lurk?

Be mindful of these sneaky sugar sources:

* Sugary drinks: Soda, juice drinks, sports drinks, and sweetened coffee beverages are loaded with added sugars. Opt for water, unsweetened tea, or black coffee instead.

* Commercially prepared desserts: Cakes, pastries, cookies, and ice cream are often high in added sugar. Choose naturally sweet fruits or homemade desserts with minimal added sugars.

* Processed snacks: Candy bars, granola bars, and chips often contain hidden sugars. Read labels carefully and choose options with lower sugar content.

Making Smart Choices:

* Satisfy your sweet tooth with naturally sweet
fruits.
* Limit sugary drinks and choose water as your
primary beverage.
* Make your own desserts at home using natural
sweeteners like honey or maple syrup in
moderation.
* Choose snacks like nuts, seeds, or plain yogurt
with low-sugar fruit toppings.

Remember:

This chapter serves as a general guideline. Your
specific needs may vary depending on your medical
history and dietary restrictions.

Part 3: Building Your Stroke Diet Meal Plan - A Roadmap to Recovery Through Food

Following a stroke, the road to recovery requires a multi-pronged approach. While medication and rehabilitation play a crucial role, what you put on your plate can significantly impact your healing journey. This section empowers you to take control of your health through the power of food.

Chapter 6: Sample Stroke-Friendly Meal Plans for Different Needs

Understanding the basic principles of a stroke diet is essential. However, individual needs and preferences can vary. This chapter provides a glimpse into what a stroke-friendly meal plan can look like for different situations:

* Sample Meal Plan for General Stroke Recovery: This plan offers a well-rounded approach for most individuals recovering from a stroke.

* Meal Plan for Individuals with Dysphagia (Swallowing Difficulties): This plan focuses on soft

and easy-to-swallow foods, catering to those with swallowing challenges.

* Diabetic-Friendly Stroke Recovery Meal Plan: This plan manages blood sugar levels while providing essential nutrients for stroke recovery.

These sample plans showcase how to incorporate the core principles of the stroke diet into practical and delicious meals, tailored to specific needs.

Chapter 7: Planning and Preparing Stroke-Friendly Meals - A Guide to Efficiency and Flavor

Eating healthy doesn't have to be complicated or time-consuming. This chapter equips you with the tools and strategies to make stroke-friendly meals a breeze, even on busy days.

* Essential Pantry Staples for the Stroke Diet: Having a well-stocked pantry lays the foundation for quick and healthy meals.

* Quick and Easy Stroke-Friendly Recipes for Busy Days: Even with a hectic schedule, you can whip up nutritious and delicious meals using these recipe ideas.

* Tips for Adapting Favorite Recipes to Fit the Stroke Diet: Don't give up on your favorite dishes! With a few simple tweaks, you can easily adapt them to be stroke-friendly.

Following these steps and utilizing the resources provided in this section, you can build a personalized and delicious stroke diet meal plan that empowers you to actively participate in your recovery journey. Remember, consistency is key. The more you embrace these healthy eating habits, the closer you'll be to achieving optimal health and well-being after a stroke.

Chapter 6: Sample Stroke-Friendly Meal Plans for Different Needs

This chapter provides a glimpse into what a stroke-friendly meal plan can look like, catering to various needs and preferences. Remember, these are just examples, and you can customize them based on your individual dietary requirements and taste preferences.

Sample Meal Plan for General Stroke Recovery

This plan offers a well-rounded approach for most individuals recovering from a stroke. It incorporates a variety of foods from the essential food groups discussed in Chapter 4.

Breakfast:

* Whole-wheat toast with scrambled eggs and sliced avocado
* Oatmeal with berries and a sprinkle of chopped nuts
* Greek yogurt with chopped fruit and a drizzle of honey

Lunch:

* Grilled chicken breast on a whole-wheat bun with lettuce, tomato, and a light vinaigrette dressing
* Lentil soup with a side salad and whole-wheat crackers
* Tuna salad sandwich on whole-wheat bread with a side of steamed vegetables

Dinner:

* Baked salmon with roasted vegetables (broccoli, carrots, sweet potatoes)
* Chicken stir-fry with brown rice and mixed vegetables
* Vegetarian chili with whole-wheat cornbread

Snacks:

* Apple slices with almond butter
* Cottage cheese with sliced vegetables
* Handful of mixed nuts and dried fruit
* Greek yogurt with a sprinkle of granola

Notes:

* Feel free to adjust portion sizes based on your individual needs.
* Choose lean protein sources and healthy fats.
* Limit processed foods and added sugars.

* Drink plenty of water throughout the day.

Meal Plan for Individuals with Dysphagia (Swallowing Difficulties)

This plan focuses on soft and easy-to-swallow foods suitable for individuals with dysphagia. Consistency and texture are crucial, and modifications may be needed depending on the severity of swallowing difficulties.

Breakfast:

* Smoothies made with yogurt, ripe banana, and berries
* Scrambled eggs with melted cheese (soft consistency)
* Mashed banana with a dollop of peanut butter

Lunch:

* Cream of vegetable soup with a side of mashed potatoes
* Well-cooked pasta with soft marinara sauce
* Scrambled tofu with chopped vegetables, served with soft whole-wheat bread

Dinner:

* Baked salmon with mashed sweet potatoes and steamed broccoli (cut into small pieces)
* Ground turkey chili with soft beans and vegetables, pureed if needed
* Chicken and rice casserole with a creamy sauce (soft consistency)

Snacks:

* Applesauce or pear sauce
* Yogurt with mashed banana
* Cottage cheese with mashed avocado
* Soft, cooked vegetables like steamed carrots or peas

Notes:

* Consult with a speech-language pathologist for specific recommendations on textures and food modifications.
* Thickening agents can be used to adjust the consistency of liquids.
* Puree or mash foods as needed to ensure safe swallowing.

Diabetic-Friendly Stroke Recovery Meal Plan

This plan manages blood sugar levels while providing the essential nutrients needed for stroke recovery. It emphasizes whole grains, lean protein, and healthy fats.

Breakfast:

* Scrambled eggs with spinach and whole-wheat toast
* Greek yogurt with berries and a sprinkle of chia seeds
* Oatmeal with chopped nuts and a drizzle of sugar-free maple syrup

Lunch:

* Grilled chicken salad with mixed greens, avocado, and a light vinaigrette dressing
* Tuna salad sandwich on whole-wheat bread with a side salad
* Lentil soup with a side of whole-wheat crackers

Dinner:

* Baked salmon with roasted Brussels sprouts and quinoa
* Turkey chili with black beans and whole-wheat cornbread (limited portion)

* Chicken stir-fry with brown rice and mixed
vegetables (limited rice portion)

Snacks:

* Apple slices with low-fat cheese
* Handful of almonds and dried cranberries
* Celery sticks with peanut butter
* Cottage cheese with chopped vegetables

Notes:

* Choose whole grains over refined grains.
* Limit sugary fruits and opt for berries with a
lower glycemic index.
* Monitor your blood sugar levels regularly.
* Consult with a registered dietitian for
personalized recommendations.

Chapter 7: Planning and Preparing Stroke-Friendly Meals - A Guide to Efficiency and Flavor

Following a stroke diet doesn't have to mean sacrificing flavor or convenience. This chapter equips you with the tools and strategies to plan, prepare, and enjoy delicious stroke-friendly meals, even on busy days.

Essential Pantry Staples for the Stroke Diet

Having a well-stocked pantry lays the foundation for quick and healthy meals. Here are some essentials to keep on hand:

* Whole Grains: Brown rice, quinoa, whole-wheat bread, and whole-wheat pasta provide sustained energy and essential fiber.

* Canned Goods: Low-sodium canned beans and lentils offer a plant-based protein source. Canned vegetables (no added salt) can be a time-saving option.

* Dried Fruits and Nuts: A handful of nuts, seeds, and dried fruits provide healthy fats, fiber, and a satisfying snack option.

* Healthy Fats: Olive oil, avocado oil, and nut butter add healthy fats and flavor to your meals.

* Spices and Herbs: Experiment with flavorful spices and herbs to add variety to your dishes without relying on added salt.

* Low-Fat Dairy: Low-fat yogurt, milk, and cheese provide calcium and vitamin D. Opt for unsweetened or minimally sweetened varieties.

* Frozen Fruits and Vegetables: Frozen options offer convenience and retain essential nutrients. Stock up on frozen berries, broccoli, spinach, and mixed vegetables.

Quick and Easy Stroke-Friendly Recipes for Busy Days

Even with a busy schedule, you can whip up nutritious and delicious meals. Here are some quick and easy recipe ideas:

Breakfast:
   * Overnight oats with yogurt, berries, and chia seeds

* Whole-wheat toast with scrambled eggs and avocado slices
* Smoothie made with Greek yogurt, banana, spinach, and almond milk

Lunch:
* Leftovers from dinner
* Tuna salad sandwich on whole-wheat bread with lettuce and tomato
* Canned bean salad with chopped vegetables and a light vinaigrette dressing

Dinner:
* Baked salmon with roasted vegetables (simple one-pan meal)
* Lentil soup with a side salad (utilizes pantry staples)
* Whole-wheat pasta with grilled chicken and a light tomato sauce

Tips for Adapting Favorite Recipes to Fit the Stroke Diet

Don't give up on your favorite dishes! With a few tweaks, you can easily adapt them to be stroke-friendly. Here are some tips:

Reduce Saturated Fat:

* Choose lean protein sources like skinless chicken or fish.
  * Trim visible fat from meats before cooking.
  * Use healthy cooking methods like grilling, baking, or steaming instead of frying.

Limit Added Sodium:
  * Rinse canned beans and vegetables to remove some of the sodium content.
  * Use herbs and spices for flavor instead of relying on salt.
  * Look for low-sodium alternatives to broths, condiments, and canned goods.

Control Portion Sizes:
  * Use measuring cups or bowls to ensure you're not overindulging.
  * Divide recipes into individual portions for easy portion control.

Healthy Swaps:
  * Replace white rice with brown rice or quinoa.
  * Use whole-wheat pasta instead of regular pasta.
  * Opt for unsweetened applesauce instead of sugar in baking recipes.

Remember:

These are just starting points. Explore my cookbooks on Stroke:

THE BEST STROKE DIET RECIPE BOOK FOR BEGINNERS and THE BEST STROKE RECOVERY DIET COOKBOOK by Eddie M.Richards.

And websites specifically designed for stroke-friendly meals. With a little creativity and these tips, you can enjoy delicious and nutritious meals that support your recovery journey.

Part 4: Stroke Diet Food Lists - Equipping Yourself for Smart Shopping

Following a stroke diet doesn't require drastic changes or complicated meal plans. In fact, with the right knowledge, you can navigate the grocery store with confidence and make informed choices that fuel your recovery. This section empowers you to become an expert on stroke-friendly foods, providing the tools you need to stock your kitchen and build a delicious and nutritious diet.

Chapter 8: Comprehensive List of Stroke-Friendly Foods by Category

Knowing which foods fall under each essential food group is the cornerstone of smart grocery shopping for a stroke diet. This chapter breaks down a comprehensive list of stroke-friendly options, categorized for your convenience: fruits, vegetables, whole grains, lean protein sources, low-fat dairy options, and healthy fats. With this knowledge at your fingertips, you can effortlessly identify the best choices while browsing the aisles.

Chapter 9: Sample Grocery Shopping List for a Stroke Diet

Getting started with a stroke diet can feel overwhelming. To ease the transition, Chapter 9 provides a sample grocery shopping list. This list serves as a blueprint, offering a variety of options within each food group. Feel free to customize it based on your preferences and the recipes you plan to prepare.

Throughout this section, you'll gain the knowledge and tools to confidently navigate the grocery store and create a stroke-friendly diet that is both delicious and supportive of your recovery journey. Let's dive into the world of stroke-friendly foods and empower yourself to make informed choices for optimal health.

Chapter 8: Comprehensive List of Stroke-Friendly Foods by Category - Your Grocery Shopping Guide

Equipping yourself with knowledge about stroke-friendly foods empowers you to make informed choices at the grocery store. This chapter serves as your guide, providing a comprehensive list of delicious and nutritious options categorized by food group. By incorporating these foods into your diet, you'll be well on your way to supporting your stroke recovery journey.

Fruits:

Fruits are a natural source of vitamins, minerals, and antioxidants, all crucial for overall health and well-being. Here are some excellent stroke-friendly fruit choices:

* Berries: Blueberries, strawberries, raspberries, and cranberries are packed with antioxidants that help combat inflammation.

* Citrus fruits: Oranges, grapefruits, and kiwifruit are rich in vitamin C, which supports immune function and promotes healing.

* Apples and Pears: These fiber-rich fruits contribute to satiety and gut health.

* Melons (watermelon, cantaloupe): Melons provide hydration and essential electrolytes, especially beneficial during hot weather.

Vegetables:

Vegetables are powerhouses of essential nutrients. They offer a variety of colors, each boasting a unique set of health benefits. Here are some stroke-friendly vegetable options to stock up on:

* Leafy Greens: Spinach, kale, and Swiss chard are rich in vitamins, minerals, and antioxidants, promoting overall health.

* Cruciferous Vegetables: Broccoli, Brussels sprouts, and cauliflower are high in fiber and contain compounds that may offer protection against chronic diseases.

* Bell Peppers: Packed with vitamin C and antioxidants, bell peppers come in various colors, adding vibrancy and flavor to your meals.

* Carrots: A classic source of beta-carotene, which converts to vitamin A, essential for vision and immune function.

* Tomatoes: A versatile vegetable rich in lycopene, an antioxidant with potential heart-protective benefits.

Whole Grains:

Whole grains are a crucial source of complex carbohydrates, providing sustained energy and dietary fiber. Here are some stroke-friendly whole-grain options:

* Brown Rice: A nutrient-rich alternative to white rice, offering more fiber, vitamins, and minerals.

* Quinoa: This protein-rich grain is a complete protein source for vegetarians and vegans, and also provides essential nutrients.

* Oats: A heart-healthy breakfast option, oats are high in soluble fiber, which helps lower cholesterol levels.

* Whole-wheat Bread and Pasta: Choose whole-wheat varieties over refined grains for

increased fiber intake and a more balanced blood sugar response.

* Barley: This chewy whole grain contains soluble fiber, beta-glucan, which may help reduce LDL ("bad") cholesterol.

Lean Protein Sources:

Lean protein is essential for building and repairing tissues, vital during the recovery process after a stroke. Here are some excellent stroke-friendly protein sources:

* Skinless Chicken and Turkey Breast: Low in fat and rich in protein, these versatile meats can be incorporated into various dishes.

* Fish: Opt for fish rich in omega-3 fatty acids, like salmon, tuna, and mackerel, which offer heart-healthy benefits.

* Beans and Lentils: An excellent plant-based protein source, beans and lentils are also high in fiber and essential nutrients.

* Tofu and Tempeh: Soy-based protein options, tofu and tempeh, are versatile and can be seasoned to complement various flavors.

* Low-Fat Yogurt: A good source of protein and calcium, low-fat yogurt can be enjoyed as a snack or incorporated into smoothies.

Low-Fat Dairy Options:

Dairy products provide essential calcium and vitamin D for bone health. Here are some stroke-friendly low-fat dairy options:

* Low-fat Milk (cow's milk or fortified plant-based milk): Choose low-fat or fat-free milk to enjoy the benefits of calcium and vitamin D without the added saturated fat.

* Low-fat Yogurt: A good source of protein and calcium, low-fat yogurt can be enjoyed as a snack or incorporated into smoothies. Opt for unsweetened or minimally sweetened varieties.

* Low-fat Cheese (cottage cheese, ricotta cheese): Lower in fat than regular cheese, these options provide protein and calcium while being lighter on calories.

Healthy Fats:

Healthy fats are essential for brain function and overall health. Here are some stroke-friendly healthy fat sources:

* Olive Oil: This versatile oil is rich in monounsaturated fats and offers numerous health benefits.

* Avocado: A creamy and delicious fruit, avocado is loaded with healthy fats, fiber, and essential nutrients.

* Nuts and Seeds: Almonds, walnuts, flaxseeds, and chia seeds are a great source of healthy fats, fiber, and protein. Enjoy them in moderation as they can be calorie-dense.

Remember:

This list is not exhaustive. Explore different varieties within each category to keep your meals interesting and flavorful. When making choices at the grocery store, prioritize fresh or frozen produce over canned options whenever possible. Canned vegetables can be a convenient option, but be sure to choose varieties packed in water or low-sodium broth to minimize sodium intake.

By incorporating these stroke-friendly foods into your diet, you'll be providing your body with the essential nutrients it needs to heal and recover after a stroke. The next chapter will take you a step further by providing a sample grocery shopping list to kickstart your stroke-friendly meal planning journey.

Chapter 9: Sample Grocery Shopping List for a Stroke Diet - A Blueprint for Success

Following a stroke diet doesn't have to be complicated. This chapter provides a sample grocery shopping list to serve as a blueprint for your stroke-friendly meal planning. Remember, this is just a starting point; feel free to customize it based on your preferences, the recipes you plan to make, and any dietary restrictions you may have.

Fruits (Choose a variety throughout the week):

* Berries (1 container)
* Apples (4)
* Bananas (4)
* Citrus fruit (grapefruit, orange) (4)

Vegetables (Select a mix of colors for a variety of nutrients):

* Leafy greens (spinach, kale) (1 bag)
* Cruciferous vegetables (broccoli, cauliflower) (1 head each)
* Bell peppers (different colors) (3)
* Carrots (5)

* Tomatoes (cherry or vine-ripened) (1 pint container)

Whole Grains (Stock up on these staples):

* Brown rice (2 bags)
* Quinoa (1 bag)
* Whole-wheat bread (1 loaf)
* Whole-wheat pasta (1 box)

Lean Protein Sources (Choose a variety throughout the week):

* Skinless chicken breasts (2 packs)
* Fish fillets (salmon, tuna) (4)
* Beans (black beans, lentils) (1-2 cans, no added salt preferred)
* Low-fat yogurt (6 individual containers)

Low-Fat Dairy Options (Select one or two options):

* Low-fat milk (cow's milk or fortified plant-based milk) (1 gallon)
* Low-fat cheese (cottage cheese, ricotta cheese) (1 block)

Healthy Fats (Incorporate these throughout the week):

* Olive oil (1 bottle)
* Avocado (2)
* Nuts and seeds (almonds, walnuts) (1 bag,
unsalted or dry-roasted)

Pantry Staples (Refer to Chapter 7 for a full list):

In addition to the fresh items above, consider
stocking your pantry with essential staples like
dried fruits, nuts, canned beans (no added salt),
whole-wheat crackers, and low-sodium broths.
These staples can be lifesavers when you need to
whip up a quick and healthy meal.

Customizing Your List:

Remember, this is just a sample. Adapt it based on
your specific needs and preferences. Here are some
ways to personalize your list:

* Portion Sizes: Adjust the quantities based on your
household size and how often you shop.

* Recipes: Plan your meals for the week and include
any specific ingredients needed for your chosen
recipes.

* Seasonal Produce: Take advantage of what's in season for the freshest and most affordable options.

* Dietary Restrictions: If you have any allergies or follow a specific diet (vegetarian, diabetic), adjust the list accordingly.

Utilizing the List:

* Print this list or keep it handy on your phone for easy reference during grocery shopping trips.
* Check off items as you add them to your cart to avoid impulse purchases.
* Don't be afraid to experiment with different options within each food group to keep your meals exciting.

By incorporating this sample list and the provided customization tips, you can create a personalized and healthy grocery shopping routine that supports your stroke recovery journey. Remember, consistency is key. The more you embrace these stroke-friendly choices, the closer you'll be to achieving optimal health and well-being.

Part 5: Recipes for Stroke Recovery - Flavorful Fuel for Your Healing Journey

Nourishing your body with delicious and nutritious meals is a cornerstone of stroke recovery. This section goes beyond the "what" to the "how," providing you with a recipe collection specifically designed to support your healing journey.

Chapter 10: Delicious and Nutritious Breakfast Recipes

Starting your day with a well-balanced breakfast sets the tone for a healthy and energetic day. This chapter offers a variety of stroke-friendly breakfast recipes that are both delicious and easy to prepare.

Chapter 11: Heart-Healthy Lunch and Dinner Options

Lunch and dinner are crucial opportunities to provide your body with the nutrients it needs for healing and recovery. This chapter features a selection of heart-healthy lunch and dinner recipes that are flavorful, satisfying, and stroke-friendly.

Chapter 12: Satisfying Snacks for Stroke Recovery

Healthy snacking can help you manage hunger pangs and maintain stable blood sugar levels. This chapter provides recipes for delicious and nutritious snacks that are perfect for a quick pick-me-up throughout the day.

Chapter 13: Easy and Flavorful Side Dishes

Side dishes can elevate a simple meal into a well-rounded and satisfying plate. This chapter offers recipes for easy and flavorful side dishes that complement your main courses while staying true to the principles of the stroke diet.

Throughout this section, you'll find recipes that are not only delicious but also:

* Easy to prepare: Many recipes require minimal prep time and cooking skills, making them perfect for busy schedules.

* Customizable: Feel free to adjust ingredients and flavors to suit your preferences and dietary needs.

* Rich in essential nutrients: Each recipe incorporates a variety of healthy ingredients to provide your body with the building blocks for healing.

With this recipe collection as your guide, you can embark on a culinary adventure that nourishes your body and delights your taste buds, all while supporting your stroke recovery journey.

Chapter 10: Delicious and Nutritious Breakfast Recipes - Fueling Your Day for Recovery

Breakfast is often referred to as the most important meal of the day, and after a stroke, it becomes even more crucial. This chapter provides a variety of delicious and nutritious breakfast recipes that are easy to prepare and gentle on your stomach, promoting optimal healing and a strong start to your day.

Recipe 1: Power Berry Smoothie

This antioxidant-rich smoothie is packed with flavor and essential nutrients.

* Ingredients:
  * 1 cup frozen berries (mixed berries, blueberries, strawberries)
  * 1 cup of low-fat, unsweetened yogurt (or plant-based yogurt)
  * ½ banana
  * ½ cup milk (dairy or fortified plant-based milk)
  * ¼ cup rolled oats
  * 1 tablespoon ground flaxseed (optional)
  * Pinch of cinnamon

* Instructions:
    1. Blend each item until it becomes creamy and smooth.
    2. Enjoy immediately.

Recipe 2: Scrambled Eggs with Spinach and Tomatoes

A classic breakfast option with a twist of leafy greens for added nutrients.

* Ingredients:
    * 2 eggs
    * 1 tablespoon low-fat milk
    * ½ cup chopped fresh spinach
    * ½ cup chopped tomatoes
    * 1 tablespoon chopped fresh chives (optional)
    * Salt and pepper to taste

* Instructions:
    1. In a bowl, whisk together eggs and milk.
    2. Heat a non-stick pan with a spritz of cooking spray.
    3. Add spinach and tomatoes to the pan and cook until softened, about 2 minutes.
    4. Pour in the egg mixture and scramble until cooked through, to your desired consistency.
    5. Season with salt, pepper, and chives (if using).

Recipe 3: Whole-Wheat Toast with Avocado and Sliced Sliced Turkey Breast

A protein-packed and satisfying option for busy mornings.

* Ingredients:
    * 1 slice whole-wheat toast
    * ½ ripe avocado, mashed
    * 2 slices lean turkey breast
    * 1 tablespoon crumbled low-fat feta cheese (optional)
    * Pinch of lemon pepper seasoning

* Instructions:
    1. Toast the whole-wheat bread to your desired crispness.
    2. Toast should be topped with mashed avocado.
    3. Top with sliced turkey breast, feta cheese (if using), and sprinkle with lemon pepper seasoning.

Recipe 4: Oatmeal with Berries and Nuts

A heart-healthy and fiber-rich breakfast option that keeps you feeling full for longer.

* Ingredients:

* ½ cup rolled oats
* 1 cup water or milk (dairy or fortified plant-based milk)
* ½ cup berries, either frozen or fresh
* ¼ cup chopped nuts, such as pecans, walnuts, and almonds
* 1 tablespoon ground flaxseed (optional)
* 1 teaspoon honey (optional)

* Instructions:
1. In a saucepan, combine oats and water or milk. Bring to a boil, then reduce heat and simmer for 5 minutes, or until oats are cooked through and creamy.
2. Stir in berries and flaxseed (if using).
3. Top with chopped nuts and drizzle with honey (if using).

Recipe 5: Chia Pudding with Mango and Coconut Flakes

A fridge-prep option perfect for mornings on the go.

* Ingredients (makes 2 servings):
* ¾ cup chia seeds
* 1 ½ cups of unsweetened almond milk (or alternative plant-based milk)
* ¼ cup chopped fresh mango

* 2 tablespoons of shredded coconut flakes
without sugar
    * 1 teaspoon vanilla extract
    * Stevia or honey to taste (optional)

* Instructions:
    1. In a jar or container, whisk together chia seeds,
almond milk, vanilla extract, and stevia or honey (if
using).
    2. Stir in chopped mango.
    3. Cover and refrigerate for at least 2 hours, or
preferably overnight, to allow the chia seeds to
thicken.
    4. In the morning, top with additional chopped
mango and coconut flakes before serving.

Recipe 6: Whole-Wheat Pancakes with Fruit Compote

A healthier take on a classic breakfast favorite.

* Ingredients (makes about 6 pancakes):
    * 1 cup whole-wheat flour
    * 1 ½ teaspoons baking powder
    * ½ teaspoon salt
    * 1 cup low-fat milk (dairy or plant-based milk)
    * 1 egg

   * 1 tablespoon melted unsalted butter or avocado oil
   * 1 teaspoon vanilla extract
   * Fresh or frozen fruit of your choice (for compote)

* Instructions:
   1. In a large bowl, whisk together the dry ingredients: whole-wheat flour, baking powder, and salt.

* In a separate bowl, whisk together the wet ingredients: milk, egg, melted butter or oil, and vanilla extract.

* Mix until just incorporated, gradually add the wet components to the dry ingredients. Don't overmix! A few lumps are okay.

* Warm up a nonstick pan or griddle that has been gently oiled over medium heat.
* Pour about 1/4 cup of batter for each pancake onto the griddle.

* Cook for 2 to 3 minutes on each side, or until well cooked and golden brown.

* While the pancakes are cooking, prepare your fruit compote (see recipe below).

Fruit Compote (makes about 1 cup):

* Ingredients:
   * 1 cup fresh or frozen fruit (berries, sliced peaches, diced apples)
   * 2 tablespoons water
   * 1 tablespoon honey or maple syrup (optional)
   * 1 teaspoon cornstarch (optional)

* Instructions:
   1. In a small saucepan, combine fruit and water.
   2. Heat to a simmer on a medium setting.
   3. If using, stir in honey or maple syrup and cornstarch (mixed with a little water to make a slurry) for a thicker consistency.
   4. Cook for 3-5 minutes, or until the fruit is softened and the sauce has thickened slightly (if using cornstarch).

Chapter 11: Heart-Healthy Lunch and Dinner Options

This chapter offers a taste of the delicious and nutritious possibilities you can explore while following a stroke-friendly diet. Each recipe prioritizes heart-healthy ingredients, essential nutrients, and ease of preparation, making them perfect for incorporating into your lunch and dinner routine.

Recipe 1: Mediterranean Quinoa Salad (Light and Refreshing)

This protein-packed salad is bursting with flavor and perfect for a light lunch or a refreshing summer dinner.

* Ingredients:
    * 1 cup cooked quinoa
    * 1 cup chopped cucumber
    * 1 cup chopped cherry tomatoes
    * ½ cup crumbled feta cheese (optional)
    * ¼ cup chopped Kalamata olives
    * ¼ cup chopped red onion
    * Handful of chopped fresh parsley
    * 2 tablespoons olive oil
    * 1 tablespoon lemon juice

* 1 teaspoon dried oregano
* Salt and pepper to taste

* Instructions:
    1. In a large bowl, combine cooked quinoa, cucumber, tomatoes, feta cheese (if using), olives, red onion, and parsley.
    2. In a separate bowl, whisk together olive oil, lemon juice, and oregano.
    3. Pour the dressing over the salad and toss to coat.
    4. Season with salt and pepper to taste.

Recipe 2: Salmon with Roasted Vegetables (Comforting and Flavorful)

This dish is a heart-healthy powerhouse, packed with omega-3 fatty acids and essential vitamins from the roasted vegetables.

* Ingredients:
    * 2 salmon fillets
    * 1 tablespoon olive oil
    * 1 teaspoon dried thyme
    * Salt and pepper to taste
    * 1 cup broccoli florets
    * 1 cup chopped red bell pepper
    * ½ cup chopped zucchini

* 1 tablespoon balsamic vinegar (optional)

* Instructions:
   1. Preheat the oven to 400°F (200°C).
   2. Toss broccoli, bell pepper, and zucchini with olive oil, salt, and pepper.
   3. Spread vegetables on a baking sheet and roast for 15-20 minutes, or until tender-crisp.
   4. Season salmon fillets with olive oil, thyme, salt, and pepper.
   5. Place salmon on a separate baking sheet or pan and bake for 10-15 minutes, or until cooked through.
   6. Drizzle with balsamic vinegar (optional) before serving and enjoy with roasted vegetables.

Recipe 3: Lentil Soup with Whole-Wheat Bread (Warm and Nourishing)

This hearty soup is packed with protein and fiber, making it a satisfying and healthy meal option.

* Ingredients:
   * 1 tablespoon olive oil
   * 1 chopped onion
   * 2 cloves garlic, minced
   * 1 cup brown lentils, rinsed
   * 4 cups vegetable broth

* 1 (14.5 oz) can diced tomatoes, undrained
* 1 cup chopped carrots
* ½ cup chopped celery
* 1 teaspoon dried thyme
* Salt and pepper to taste
* Slices of whole-wheat bread for serving

* Instructions:
    1. Heat olive oil in a large pot over medium heat.
    2. Add onion and garlic and cook until softened, about 5 minutes.
    3. Stir in lentils, vegetable broth, diced tomatoes, carrots, celery, and thyme.
    4. Bring to a boil, then reduce heat and simmer for 30-35 minutes, or until lentils are tender.
    5. Season with salt and pepper to taste.
    6. Serve hot with a slice of whole-wheat bread for dipping.

Recipe 4: Turkey Burgers with Sweet Potato Fries (Satisfying and Fun)

This recipe offers a healthier twist on a classic favorite, perfect for a satisfying and flavorful dinner.

* Ingredients (makes 2 burgers):
    * ½ pound ground turkey

* ¼ cup chopped onion
* ¼ cup chopped bell pepper
* 1 tablespoon chopped fresh parsley
* 1 egg, beaten
* ½ cup whole-wheat breadcrumbs
* Salt and pepper to taste
* 1 sweet potato, cut into wedges
* 1 tablespoon olive oil

* Instructions:
    1. Preheat the oven to 400°F (200°C).
    2. In a large bowl, combine ground turkey, onion, bell pepper, parsley, egg, breadcrumbs, salt, and pepper.
    3. Form the mixture into two equal patties.
    4. Toss sweet potato wedges with olive oil and spread on a baking sheet.
    5. Bake sweet potato wedges for 20-25 minutes, flipping halfway through.

* Heat a lightly greased skillet over medium heat.
* Cook the turkey burgers for 4-5 minutes per side, or until cooked through.
* Serve the turkey burgers on whole-wheat buns (optional) with baked sweet potato fries and your favorite toppings.

Recipe 5: Vegetarian Black Bean Chili (Flavorful and Protein-Packed)

This chili is a vegetarian delight, brimming with protein and fiber from black beans and kidney beans.

* Ingredients:
    * 1 tablespoon olive oil
    * 1 chopped onion
    * 2 cloves garlic, minced
    * 1 green bell pepper, chopped
    * 1 (15 oz) can diced tomatoes, undrained
    * 1 (15 oz) can black beans, rinsed and drained
    * 1 (15 oz) can kidney beans, rinsed and drained
    * 4 cups vegetable broth
    * 1 tablespoon chili powder
    * 1 teaspoon ground cumin
    * ½ teaspoon dried oregano
    * Salt and pepper to taste
    * Optional toppings: chopped avocado, shredded cheese, low-fat sour cream

* Instructions:
    1. Heat olive oil in a large pot or Dutch oven over medium heat.
    2. Add onion, garlic, and bell pepper and cook until softened, about 5 minutes.

3. Stir in diced tomatoes, black beans, kidney beans, vegetable broth, chili powder, cumin, and oregano.

4. Bring to a boil, then reduce heat and simmer for 20-25 minutes, or until flavors meld.

5. Season with salt and pepper to taste.

6. Serve hot with your favorite toppings, such as chopped avocado, shredded cheese, or low-fat sour cream.

Recipe 6: Chicken Stir-Fry with Brown Rice (Easy and Customizable)

This quick and easy stir-fry is a great way to incorporate lean protein and vegetables into your diet.

* Ingredients:
    * 1 tablespoon cornstarch
    * 2 tablespoons soy sauce (low-sodium preferred)
    * 1 tablespoon rice vinegar
    * 1 tablespoon honey
    * 1 tablespoon water
    * 1 pound boneless, skinless chicken breasts, thinly sliced
    * 1 tablespoon olive oil
    * 1 cup broccoli florets
    * ½ cup sliced red bell pepper

* ½ cup chopped carrots
* 2 cloves garlic, minced
* Cooked brown rice, for serving

* Instructions:
1. In a small bowl, whisk together cornstarch, soy sauce, rice vinegar, honey, and water.
2. Heat olive oil in a large skillet or wok over medium-high heat.
3. Add chicken and cook until browned and cooked through, about 5 minutes.
4. Stir in broccoli, bell pepper, and carrots, and cook for an additional 3-4 minutes, or until vegetables are tender-crisp.
5. Add the prepared sauce to the pan and cook until slightly thickened, about 1-2 minutes.
6. Serve chicken stir-fry over cooked brown rice.

Chapter 12: Satisfying Snacks for Stroke Recovery - Delicious Bites to Power Your Healing

Managing hunger pangs and keeping your blood sugar levels stable is crucial for stroke recovery. This chapter offers a delightful selection of snack recipes specifically designed to be both satisfying and stroke-friendly. Each recipe prioritizes heart-healthy ingredients, providing you with essential nutrients for optimal healing throughout the day.

Smart Snacking for Stroke Recovery:

* Portion Control: Keep serving sizes in mind to avoid overeating. Aim for small, satisfying portions to curb hunger without compromising your overall dietary goals.

* Nutrient Balance: Strive for a combination of protein, fiber, and healthy fats in your snacks. This well-rounded approach keeps you feeling full for longer and provides your body with the building blocks it needs for recovery.

* Sodium and Saturated Fat Awareness: Choose snacks that are lower in sodium and saturated fat to promote cardiovascular health.

Delicious and Nutritious Snack Inspiration:

1. Cinnamon Apple Nachos: (Unique and Refreshing)

* Ingredients:
    * 1 medium apple, thinly sliced
    * 1/4 cup low-fat ricotta cheese
    * 1 tablespoon chopped walnuts
    * 1/2 teaspoon ground cinnamon

* Instructions:
    1. Arrange apple slices on a plate.
    2. Top with dollops of ricotta cheese.
    3. Sprinkle it with chopped walnuts and cinnamon.
    4. Enjoy this delightful combination of sweet, creamy, and crunchy textures.

2. Mini Bell Pepper Boats with Guacamole: (Light and Flavorful)

* Ingredients:
    * 1 red bell pepper, cut into wedges

* 1/2 cup prepared guacamole
* Chopped fresh cilantro (optional)

* Instructions:
1. Seed and slice the bell pepper into wedges or small boats.
2. Fill each boat with a dollop of guacamole.
3. Garnish with chopped cilantro (optional) for an extra burst of flavor.
4. Enjoy this refreshing and vibrant snack that's packed with vitamins and healthy fats.

3. Frozen Yogurt Bites with Berries: (Sweet and Satisfying)

* Ingredients:
* 1 cup plain Greek yogurt
* 1/4 cup mashed berries (blueberries, raspberries)
* 1 tablespoon honey (optional)

* Instructions:
1. In a small bowl, combine Greek yogurt and mashed berries.
2. If desired, add a touch of honey for sweetness.
3. Spoon the mixture into a silicone mold or ice cube tray.

4. Freeze for several hours, or until solid.

5. Enjoy these frozen yogurt bites for a delicious and cool way to satisfy a sweet tooth.

4. Edamame Salad with Edamame, Vegetables, and Vinaigrette: (Protein-Packed and Crunchy)

   * Ingredients:
      * 1 cup shelled edamame, cooked
      * 1/2 cup chopped cucumber
      * 1/4 cup chopped red onion
      * 2 tablespoons crumbled feta cheese (optional)
      * 2 tablespoons light vinaigrette dressing

   * Instructions:
      1. In a bowl, combine cooked edamame, chopped cucumber, and red onion.

      2. Crumble feta cheese over the salad (optional).

      3. Drizzle with light vinaigrette dressing and toss to coat.

      4. Enjoy this protein-rich and crunchy salad for a satisfying snack.

5. Homemade Trail Mix with a Twist: (Customizable and Nutritious)

* Ingredients:
    * 1/2 cup dry whole-grain cereal squares
    * 1/4 cup roasted almonds
    * 1/4 cup dried cranberries
    * 1/4 cup pumpkin seeds
    * 1 tablespoon dark chocolate chips (optional)

* Instructions:
1. In a bowl, combine dry cereal squares, almonds, cranberries, and pumpkin seeds.
2. For an extra touch of indulgence, add dark chocolate chips (optional).
3. This recipe allows you to customize the ingredients based on your preferences, ensuring a delicious and satisfying snack mix.

6. Spicy Roasted Chickpeas: (Crunchy and Flavorful)

* Ingredients:
    * 1 can chickpeas, rinsed and drained
    * 1 tablespoon olive oil
    * 1/2 teaspoon chili powder
    * 1/4 teaspoon smoked paprika
    * 1/4 teaspoon ground cumin
    * Pinch of cayenne pepper (optional)
    * Salt and pepper to taste

* Instructions:

1. Preheat the oven to 400°F (200°C).

2. Pat chickpeas dry with a paper towel.

3. In a bowl, toss chickpeas with olive oil, chili powder, paprika, cumin, cayenne pepper (if using), salt, and pepper.

4. Spread chickpeas on a baking sheet and roast for 20-25 minutes, or until golden brown and crispy.

5. Let cool slightly before enjoying this flavorful and crunchy snack that is perfect for satisfying cravings while managing your sodium intake.

Chapter 13: Easy and Flavorful Side Dishes

This chapter offers a taste of the delicious and nutritious possibilities when it comes to side dishes for a stroke-friendly diet. Each recipe prioritizes ease of preparation, essential nutrients, and flavor, making them perfect additions to your meals.

Recipe 1: Lemon Herb Roasted Asparagus (Roasted Vegetables):

This simple yet elegant side dish allows the natural flavor of asparagus to shine.

* Ingredients:
    * 1 pound asparagus spears, trimmed
    * 1 tablespoon olive oil
    * 1 teaspoon lemon zest
    * ½ teaspoon dried thyme
    * Salt and pepper to taste

* Instructions:
    1. Preheat the oven to 400°F (200°C).
    2. Toss asparagus spears with olive oil, lemon zest, thyme, salt, and pepper.
    3. Spread asparagus on a baking sheet in a single layer.

4. Roast for 10-12 minutes, or until tender-crisp, flipping halfway through.

Recipe 2: Greek Chickpea Salad (Quick and Easy Salads):

This protein-packed salad is bursting with Mediterranean flavors and perfect for a light and refreshing side dish.

* Ingredients:
    * 1 can (15 oz) chickpeas, rinsed and drained
    * 1 cucumber, chopped
    * 1 tomato, chopped
    * ½ cup crumbled feta cheese (optional)
    * ¼ cup chopped red onion
    * ¼ cup Kalamata olives, halved
    * 2 tablespoons olive oil
    * 1 tablespoon lemon juice
    * 1 teaspoon dried oregano
    * Salt and pepper to taste

* Instructions:
    1. In a large bowl, combine chickpeas, cucumber, tomato, feta cheese (if using), red onion, and olives.
    2. In a separate bowl, whisk together olive oil, lemon juice, and oregano.

3. Pour the dressing over the salad and toss to coat.

4. Season with salt and pepper to taste.

Recipe 3: Quinoa with Roasted Butternut Squash (Flavorful Grains):

This warm and comforting dish combines the fluffy texture of quinoa with the sweetness of roasted butternut squash.

* Ingredients:
    * 1 cup quinoa, rinsed
    * 1 ½ cups vegetable broth
    * 1 medium butternut squash, peeled and cubed
    * 1 tablespoon olive oil
    * ½ teaspoon ground cinnamon
    * ¼ teaspoon ground nutmeg
    * Salt and pepper to taste

* Instructions:
    1. Preheat the oven to 400°F (200°C).
    2. Toss butternut squash cubes with olive oil, cinnamon, nutmeg, salt, and pepper.
    3. Spread squash on a baking sheet and roast for 20-25 minutes, or until tender-crisp.
    4. In a saucepan, combine rinsed quinoa and vegetable broth.

5. Bring to a boil, then reduce heat, cover, and simmer for 15 minutes, or until quinoa is cooked and fluffy.

6. Fluff the quinoa with a fork and stir in roasted butternut squash.

7. Season with additional salt and pepper to taste (optional).

Recipe 4: Creamy Carrot and Parsnip Mash (Mashed Delights):

This recipe offers a healthy twist on mashed potatoes. Combining carrots and parsnips creates a naturally sweet and creamy side dish.

* Ingredients:
   * 2 pounds carrots and parsnips, peeled and chopped
   * ½ cup low-fat milk (or plant-based milk)
   * 1 tablespoon unsalted butter
   * Salt and pepper to taste
   * Fresh chopped chives (optional, for garnish)

* Instructions:
   1. In a large pot, cover chopped carrots and parsnips with water and bring to a boil.
   2. Reduce heat and simmer for 15-20 minutes, or until tender.

3. Drain the water and return the vegetables to the pot.

4. Using a hand mixer or potato masher, mash the vegetables until smooth.

5. Gradually stir in milk and butter until desired consistency is reached.

6. Season with salt and pepper to taste.

7. Garnish with fresh chopped chives (optional) and serve.

Recipe 5: Balsamic Glazed Green Beans with Toasted Almonds (Quick and Easy Salads):

This quick and flavorful salad offers a delightful combination of textures and tastes.

* Ingredients:
    * 1 pound fresh green beans, trimmed
    * 1 tablespoon olive oil
    * 2 tablespoons balsamic vinegar
    * 1 tablespoon honey
    * ¼ cup sliced almonds, toasted
    * Salt
    * Pepper to taste

* Instructions:
    1. In a large pot of boiling water, blanch the green beans for 3-4 minutes, or until tender-crisp.

2. Drain the beans and rinse under cold water to stop the cooking process.

3. In a large skillet, heat olive oil over medium heat.

4. Add balsamic vinegar and honey, whisking to combine and scraping up any browned bits from the bottom of the pan.

5. Bring the mixture to a simmer and cook for 2-3 minutes, or until slightly thickened.

6. Add the blanched green beans to the pan and toss to coat them in the balsamic glaze.

7. Season with salt and pepper to taste.

8. Remove from heat and stir in toasted almonds.

9. Serve warm or at room temperature.

Recipe 6: Garlic Parmesan Zucchini Noodles (Roasted Vegetables):

This recipe offers a delicious low-carb alternative to pasta. Spiralized zucchini is roasted with garlic and parmesan cheese for a flavorful and satisfying side dish.

* Ingredients:
    * 2 medium zucchini, spiralized into noodles
    * 1 tablespoon olive oil
    * 2 cloves garlic, minced
    * ¼ cup grated Parmesan cheese

* Salt and pepper to taste
* Fresh chopped parsley (optional, for garnish)

* Instructions:
   1. Preheat the oven to 400°F (200°C).
   2. In a large bowl, toss zucchini noodles with olive oil, garlic, and salt and pepper.
   3. Spread the zucchini noodles on a baking sheet in a single layer.
   4. Roast for 15-20 minutes, or until tender-crisp, flipping halfway through.
   5. Remove from the oven and sprinkle with Parmesan cheese.
   6. Broil for an additional 1-2 minutes, or until the cheese is melted and slightly golden brown.
   7. Garnish with fresh chopped parsley (optional) and serve.

Part 6: Living with the Stroke Diet - Maintaining a Healthy and Fulfilling Journey

Following a stroke, a healthy diet plays a crucial role in your recovery. Part 5 has equipped you with delicious recipes and essential information for preparing nutritious meals at home. However, navigating social situations and maintaining motivation can be challenging.

Part 6 delves into these aspects of living with a stroke diet, offering valuable guidance and support:

Chapter 14: Dining Out on the Stroke Diet: Making Healthy Choices: Learn valuable strategies for making informed decisions when dining out, ensuring your restaurant meals align with your stroke-friendly diet.

Chapter 15: Maintaining Motivation and Overcoming Challenges: Explore strategies to stay motivated and overcome challenges that may arise throughout your dietary journey. Discover tips for managing cravings, incorporating variety into your meals, and staying positive along the way.

Chapter 16: Additional Resources and Support for Stroke Recovery: This chapter provides valuable resources and support options to empower you on your stroke recovery journey. It may include information on support groups, online communities, and healthcare professionals who can provide additional guidance and encouragement.

Living with a stroke diet is not just about restrictions, it's about embracing a healthy lifestyle that promotes recovery and well-being. Part 6 equips you with the tools and knowledge to navigate challenges, maintain motivation, and find joy in the food you eat. Let's embark on this journey together, creating a sustainable and fulfilling dietary approach for a healthier you.

Chapter 14: Dining Out on the Stroke Diet: Making Healthy Choices

Enjoying a meal with friends and family is a cherished part of life. But following a stroke diet, navigating restaurant menus can feel daunting. Fear not! This chapter equips you with valuable strategies to make informed decisions and enjoy delicious meals while staying true to your dietary goals.

Planning for Success:

* Research Restaurant Menus: Many restaurants offer menus online. Browse through options beforehand to identify dishes that align with your stroke-friendly diet. Look for keywords like "grilled," "baked," "broiled," and "steamed" for healthier cooking methods.

* Consider Portion Sizes: Restaurant portions tend to be larger than typical home-cooked meals. Split an entree with a friend or opt for an appetizer as your main course.

* Communicate with Your Server: Don't hesitate to explain your dietary needs to your server. They can

help you with ingredient modifications or recommend suitable dishes.

Menu Maneuvering:

* Protein Powerhouses: Prioritize lean protein sources like grilled chicken, fish, or tofu. Avoid fried options and opt for skinless chicken or fish whenever possible.

* Fiber Fantastic Choices: Incorporate fiber-rich vegetables into your meal. Steamed broccoli, roasted asparagus, or a side salad with minimal dressing are excellent choices.

* Healthy Fat Focus: Choose dishes with healthy fats like olive oil or avocado. Avoid creamy sauces or dishes laden with butter.

* Sodium Savvy Selections: Be mindful of sodium content. Opt for grilled or baked dishes instead of salty options like cured meats or processed foods.

* Sweet Treat Strategies: Desserts can be tricky. Consider sharing a dessert with a friend or opting for a fruit plate for a lighter and more nutritious option.

Making Modifications:

* Don't be shy about requesting modifications: Many restaurants can accommodate minor adjustments. Ask for sauces on the side, dressings held, or cheese omitted. This allows you to control the amount of sodium, fat, and added sugars in your meal.

* Embrace Flavorful Alternatives: Enhance your dish with herbs and spices instead of relying on salty seasonings.

Remember:

* Enjoy the Company: Dining out is about more than just the food. Savor the company of loved ones and focus on creating lasting memories.

* It's Okay to Say No: Don't feel pressured to order something that doesn't align with your dietary needs. There's no shame in asking for a simple grilled chicken or fish with steamed vegetables.

By following these tips and embracing a proactive approach, you can navigate restaurant menus with confidence and enjoy delicious and healthy meals while dining out on your stroke-recovery journey.

Chapter 15: Maintaining Motivation and Overcoming Challenges - Sticking with Your Stroke-Friendly Diet

Following a stroke diet is an essential part of your recovery journey. However, staying motivated and overcoming challenges can be difficult. This chapter explores strategies to help you maintain focus, navigate cravings, and create a sustainable and enjoyable dietary approach.

Staying Motivated for Long-Term Success:

* Focus on the "Why":* Remind yourself of the reasons behind your dietary changes. Improved health, increased energy levels, and a better quality of life are all powerful motivators.

* Set Realistic Goals: Don't overwhelm yourself with drastic changes. Set small, achievable goals like incorporating one additional serving of vegetables per day or swapping sugary drinks for water. Celebrate your successes along the way!

* Find an Accountability Partner: Enlist the support of a friend, family member, or healthcare professional to help you stay on track. Sharing your goals and progress can boost your motivation.

* Make it Fun!: Explore new recipes, experiment with different flavors, and find healthy dishes you genuinely enjoy. Cooking can be a fun and rewarding activity.

Taming Cravings and Making Smart Choices:

* Plan Ahead: Having healthy snacks readily available can help curb cravings for unhealthy options. Stock your pantry with fruits, vegetables, and whole-grain crackers.

* Identify Your Triggers: Recognize situations or emotions that trigger unhealthy cravings. Develop coping mechanisms like taking a walk, drinking water, or engaging in a relaxing activity.

* Don't Deprive Yourself: Allow yourself occasional treats in moderation. A small piece of dark chocolate or a square of whole-wheat toast with a light spread can satisfy cravings without derailing your progress.

* Mindful Eating: Pay attention to hunger cues and eat slowly. Savor the flavors and textures of your food, allowing your body to register fullness signals.

Overcoming Challenges and Finding Support:

* Expect Setbacks: Everyone experiences occasional slip-ups. Don't beat yourself up – learn from the experience and get back on track.

* Celebrate Non-Scale Victories: Focus on progress beyond weight loss. Increased energy levels, improved blood pressure, or better sleep are all positive outcomes of a healthy diet.

* Seek Support: Don't hesitate to seek support from your healthcare team, a registered dietitian, or a support group for stroke survivors. They can offer valuable guidance and encouragement.

Remember, a healthy diet is a lifelong journey, not a temporary fix. By incorporating these strategies, you can overcome challenges, stay motivated, and create a sustainable and fulfilling dietary approach for your stroke recovery and beyond. Embrace the positive changes you're making for your health, and enjoy the delicious and nutritious journey ahead!

Chapter 16: Additional Resources and Support for Stroke Recovery - Empowering Your Journey

Following a stroke, the path to recovery requires a multifaceted approach. A healthy diet is a crucial component, but it's just one piece of the puzzle. This chapter empowers you by providing valuable resources and support options to enhance your overall well-being.

Building Your Support Network:

* Healthcare Professionals: Your primary care physician, neurologist, and rehabilitation team are invaluable resources. They can monitor your progress, answer your questions, and provide personalized guidance for your stroke recovery journey.

* Registered Dietitians: These specialists can create a personalized stroke-friendly meal plan tailored to your specific needs and preferences. They can also offer guidance on grocery shopping, healthy cooking techniques, and managing cravings.

* Support Groups: Connecting with other stroke survivors can be incredibly helpful. Sharing

experiences, offering encouragement, and learning from each other can be a powerful source of support. Look for online communities or local support groups specifically for stroke survivors.

* Stroke Association and Similar Organizations: National organizations dedicated to stroke awareness and recovery offer a wealth of resources. These organizations often provide educational materials, online communities, and support programs specifically designed for stroke survivors and their caregivers. Some examples include:
    * The National Stroke Association (https://www.stroke.org/en/)

    * The American Heart Association (https://www.heart.org/)

Additional Resources for a Holistic Approach:

* Physical Therapy: Rehabilitation exercises prescribed by a physical therapist can help improve mobility, strength, and coordination.

* Occupational Therapy: Occupational therapists can assist you in regaining independence with daily living activities like dressing, bathing, and meal preparation.

* Speech Therapy: If you are experiencing speech or language difficulties after a stroke, speech therapy can help improve communication skills.

* Mental Health Support: Stroke can impact your emotional well-being. Don't hesitate to seek support from a therapist or counselor to manage stress, anxiety, or depression.

Remember:

* Empowerment Through Knowledge: Educate yourself about stroke recovery to make informed decisions about your care. Utilize the resources listed above to learn more about stroke, healthy living, and managing your condition.

* Embrace a Holistic Approach: Stroke recovery encompasses various aspects of your life. Focus on physical well-being, mental health, and emotional support to create a comprehensive recovery plan.

* Advocate for Yourself: Don't be afraid to ask questions and voice your concerns to your healthcare team. You are an active participant in your recovery journey.

By utilizing the resources and support systems available, you can empower yourself to achieve optimal health and well-being throughout your stroke recovery journey. Remember, you are not alone. With a dedicated network of support and a commitment to a healthy lifestyle, you can navigate challenges and create a brighter future.

Appendix

Measurement Equivalents and Conversion Charts

Following recipes precisely is crucial for successful cooking, especially when managing a specific diet. This section provides conversion charts to ensure you have the correct measurements for your stroke-friendly recipes:

Volume Conversions:

Unit	Equivalent
1 teaspoon (tsp)	3 teaspoons (tsp) = 1 tablespoon (tbsp)
1 tablespoon (tbsp)	16 tablespoons (tbsp) = 1 cup (cup)
1 cup (cup)	2 cups (cup) = 1 pint (pt)
1 cup (cup)	4 cups (cup) = 1 quart (qt)
1 liter (L)	1 liter (L) = 4 cups (cup)
1 milliliter (mL)	1 milliliter (mL) = 1 teaspoon (tsp)

Weight Conversions:

| Unit | Equivalent |

|---|---|
1 ounce (oz)	16 ounces (oz) = 1 pound (lb)
1 gram (g)	28 grams (g) = 1 ounce (oz)
1 kilogram (kg)	1 kilogram (kg) = 2.2 pounds (lb)

Temperature Conversions:

Fahrenheit (°F)	Celsius (°C)
200°F	93°C
250°F	121°C
300°F	149°C
350°F	177°C
400°F	204°C

Food Safety Guidelines for Stroke Patients

Following proper food safety practices is essential for everyone, but especially for those with compromised immune systems, which can be a consequence of stroke. Here are some key guidelines to follow:

* Cleanliness: Wash your hands thoroughly with soap and warm water for at least 20 seconds before and after handling food.

* Sanitize Surfaces: Clean and disinfect countertops, cutting boards, and utensils before and after preparing food.

* Proper Storage: Store raw meat, poultry, and seafood in sealed containers on the bottom shelf of your refrigerator to prevent cross-contamination.

* Cooking Temperatures: Cook meat, poultry, and fish to their recommended internal temperatures to ensure harmful bacteria are destroyed. Use a food thermometer to check for safe temperatures.

* Refrigerate Leftovers: Promptly refrigerate any leftovers within 2 hours of cooking. Reheat leftovers to an internal temperature of 165°F (74°C) before serving.

* Beware of Expired Foods: Always check expiration dates and avoid consuming food past its designated shelf life.

By following these guidelines, you can minimize the risk of foodborne illness and ensure the safety of your meals throughout your stroke recovery journey.

Glossary of Stroke-Related Terms

Understanding medical terminology can be empowering and help you actively participate in your healthcare. Here's a glossary of some common stroke-related terms you may encounter:

* Stroke: A sudden interruption of blood flow to the brain, resulting in the death of brain cells.

* Ischemic Stroke: The most common type of stroke, caused by a blood clot blocking an artery in the brain.

* Hemorrhagic Stroke: Caused by a weakened blood vessel in the brain that bursts and bleeds.

* Transient Ischemic Attack (TIA): A "mini-stroke" caused by a temporary blockage of blood flow to the brain. Symptoms typically resolve within 24 hours.

* Atherosclerosis: Hardening and narrowing of the arteries due to plaque buildup.

* Aphasia: A language disorder that can make it difficult to speak, understand, read, or write.

* Dysarthria: Difficulty speaking due to weakness or paralysis in the muscles used for speech.

* Aphasia: A language disorder that can make it difficult to speak, understand, read, or write.

* Paralysis: Loss of muscle function in a part of the body.

* Rehabilitation: A program to help regain skills lost after a stroke, such as mobility, speech, and daily living activities.

This glossary provides a starting point. Don't hesitate to ask your healthcare team for clarification on any unfamiliar terms you encounter. By understanding your condition, you can make informed decisions about your stroke recovery journey.